VEGAN DESSERT COOKBOOK FOR SENIORS

Tasty & Nutritious Treats for Healthy Aging.

Elsa Lindsay

TABLE OF CONTENTS

INTRODUCTION

In the small town of Beaver Corners, Martha Baker was well-known for her delightful baking skills. People would flock to her bakery for her famous vegan cookies. When Martha began to get older, she knew she wanted to share her passions with others. At 76-years-old, Martha decided to create a vegan dessert cookbook specifically designed for seniors. She knew that banishing sugar, flour, and eggs from her recipes used to be challenging. But with her newfound knowledge of vegan ingredients, she was determined to make vegan desserts that were simple and delicious.

The cookbook was an immediate success, with older generations across the state discovering how to bake delicious vegan desserts. Martha's recipes were low in sugar, with alternatives like pureed dates and applesauce. She mixed oats, nut butters and banana for a yummy, non-dairy alternative to traditional cookie recipes. Her vegan copycat pack of carrot cake and pumpkin muffins were a hit. Martha included helpful advice for all her plant-based desserts, including storing tips and serving suggestions. The cookbook even opened up the entire world of vegan cooking to her readers. Martha was so proud of her cookbook. It was a testament to her love of vegan baking and her desire to share her knowledge with seniors across the country.

Today, her vegan dessert cookbook for seniors is one of the most-loved cookbooks in the bakeries of Beaver Corners. Vegan desserts can be a delicious and nutritious way to satisfy your sweet tooth. They are typically made without any animal products no eggs, dairy, or honey which makes them well-suited for those following a plant-based diet or for those looking to reduce their intake of animal products. With a bit of creativity and the right ingredients, you can create vegan desserts that are just as flavorful and indulgent as their traditional counterparts.

Vegan desserts are typically made using various plant-based ingredients, such as nuts, nut butters, coconut oil and coconut cream, plant-based milks, various flours (such as almond or coconut flour), and natural sweeteners (such as pure maple syrup or coconut sugar). These ingredients can come together to create an array of sweet treats, such as cakes, cupcakes, cookies, brownies, ice cream, puddings, pies, and more. And in some cases, vegan baking can be even healthier than traditional baking, as you can opt for whole grain flours, natural sweeteners, and more nutrient-rich ingredients that offer added nutritional benefits.

If you're looking to try your hand at vegan baking, the best place to start is by exploring classic recipes and experimenting with alternative ingredients to make them vegan-friendly. Once you've mastered the basics and felt more confident, you can go beyond traditional desserts and start creating your own vegan treats. Have fun and enjoy the process, and you'll be surprised at the delicious vegan desserts you will create.

Chapter *1*

Vegan Cupcakes

Vegan cupcakes are the perfect treat for those who are looking to grab a sweet snack without sacrificing their vegan lifestyle. These treats can be made with just a few simple ingredient swaps and some creativity, making them a great choice for those looking for a delicious treat but also for those with dietary needs or restrictions.

Vegan cupcakes can vary greatly in their ingredients, with some recipes calling for vegan-friendly ingredients like coconut oil, almond flour, and even flax egg. Other recipes may require substitutes for traditional egg and dairy products, such as vegan-friendly cream cheese. As for the sweetness in these cupcakes, pureed dates and maple syrup are excellent vegan-friendly substitutes for sugar! Vegan cupcakes are incredibly versatile, as they can be decorated with anything from sprinkles to vegan-friendly frosting, made with vegan margarine, vegan cream cheese, and a mix of vegan-friendly flavorings.

Additionally, vegan cupcakes can be loaded with all types of vegan-friendly goodies like fresh fruit, nuts, seeds, and even vegan chocolate chips! With so many different ingredients and ways to customize them, vegan cupcakes are sure to be a hit among vegans and non-vegans alike. No matter what occasion, vegan cupcakes will make an amazing treat for those looking to eat vegan-friendly snacks. Not only are they delicious and sweet, but they are also good for the environment, support animal rights, and are better for one's health. So why not give them a try? Enjoy and have fun baking your own vegan cupcake recipes at home!

Vanilla cupcakes are a classic sweet treat that can be enjoyed for any occasion. They are deliciously moist and soft, thanks to the combination of vanilla extract, unsalted butter, sugar, eggs, and all-purpose flour. Vanilla cupcakes can be topped with a luscious layer of buttercream frosting or a tangy cream cheese frosting for an extra level of sweet indulgence. The fluffy and airy texture of the cupcakes' pairs perfectly with the flavorful frostings, making them an irresistible treat that anyone can enjoy. There are countless options when it comes to aesthetic. From simple sprinkles to elegant fondant designs, Vanilla cupcakes can be decorated in a number of ways to suit any event or gathering. They make a wonderful dessert option for birthdays, baby showers, and weddings. With just a few simple ingredients, you can make a batch of delicious Vanilla cupcakes that will make any occasion even more special.

To bake the perfect batch of Vanilla cupcakes, start by preheating the oven and line a muffin tray with cupcake holders. Cream the butter and sugar together until light and fluffy, then add the eggs one at a time and mix until combined. Slowly add the dry ingredients: flour and baking powder while continuously stirring. Once everything is well combined, add the vanilla extract and stir until ingredients are thoroughly mixed. Next, spoon the batter into the cupcake holders and bake for 15-20 minutes, or until a toothpick inserted into one cupcake comes out clean. Let cupcakes cool before adding the desired frosting and decoration. Enjoy!

1.2

Chocolate cupcakes are a classic go-to delicacy for all sweet-tooth cravings. Rich and incredibly moist, even a small bite of a chocolate cupcake can be a luxurious experience. Each cupcake is delicately topped with a mound of creamy chocolate frosting, making it impossible to resist. The aroma of fresh chocolate cupcakes wafting in the air can entice even the most disciplined of eaters. Each bite of a chocolate cupcake brings a burst of flavor, beginning with the light and airy chocolate cake base. An ever-so-slight hint of sweetness floods the taste buds as a luscious cocoa flavor quickly yields to notes of rich, creamy chocolate. Followed by a subtle blend of spices, such as a hint of nutmeg or clove, each bite yields an out-of-this-world delight. The truly special part comes with the addition of the luxurious chocolate frosting.

Swirled in a thick mountain, the creamy milk chocolate frosting adds a delightful sweet and silky-smooth feel to the cupcake. When all combined, a properly chocolate cupcake is an experience like no other. Chocolate cupcakes are a fantastic addition to any party or gathering. No matter the occasion, they're sure to be a crowd pleaser. From birthdays, holidays and graduations to just enjoying a good treat, everyone can count on chocolate cupcakes to satisfy their sweet tooth cravings. Don't wait another minute, indulge your cravings head on with a moist, creamy and mouth-watering chocolate cupcake. Your taste buds will thank you.

Lemon cupcakes are a classic springtime treat. With a fluffy, buttery base and a tart and sweet lemon zest frosting, they are sure to please any palate. Perfect for a baby shower, bridal shower, or an afternoon tea, these cupcakes are sure to be a crowd pleaser. To make them, all you need is butter, sugar, vanilla extract, eggs, all-purpose flour, baking powder, salt, milk, and freshly-squeezed lemon juice and zest. Start by creaming the butter and sugar until light in color and fluffy in texture. Then, add the vanilla extract, eggs, and milk and mix until incorporated. In a separate bowl, combine the flour, baking powder, and salt and slowly beat it into the wet ingredients. Fill cupcake liners three-quarters full with the batter and bake in the oven for 18-20 minutes at 350ºF. Once cooled, they're ready to frost! For the frosting, you'll need butter, confectioners' sugar, fresh lemon juice, and zest. Simply beat the butter until light in color and fluffy in texture, then add the remaining ingredients one at a time until it reaches a spreadable consistency. Top the cooled cupcakes with a generous scoop and a decorative sprinkle of lemon zest. These lemon cupcakes are sure to be a hit; their sweet, tart, and fluffy goodness will put a smile on anyone's face. Enjoy!

Chapter 2

Vegan Pies

Vegan pies have become a popular and delectable culinary trend, appealing not only to vegans but also to those looking to explore plant-based alternatives. These pies are entirely free of animal products, making them an ethical and environmentally conscious choice. Whether you're a seasoned vegan or simply interested in trying something new, vegan pies offer a wide array of flavors and textures that are sure to satisfy your taste buds.

One of the primary challenges in creating vegan pies is replacing traditional animal-based ingredients such as butter, eggs, and dairy. However, thanks to innovative and resourceful culinary techniques, bakers have devised a plethora of creative substitutions that yield excellent results. The crust, which is a fundamental component of any pie, is typically made with plant-based fats like coconut oil, vegetable shortening, or non-dairy margarine instead of butter. These fats provide the essential flakiness and texture needed for a perfect pie crust. Additionally, using alternative types of flour, such as almond, oat, or chickpea flour, ensures that the crust remains free of animal products.

For the pie filling, the possibilities are virtually endless. Fruit-based pies, like apple, blueberry, or cherry, are popular choices and can easily be adapted to a vegan version. The filling can be sweetened with natural sweeteners like maple syrup, agave nectar, or coconut sugar. Other creative options include vegan pumpkin pie, pecan pie, and even vegan chocolate silk pie, made with silken tofu as a creamy base. Savory vegan pies are also gaining popularity, offering a satisfying and hearty meal option. For example, a classic vegan pot pie might include a rich vegetable and lentil filling, complemented by a savory gravy made from vegetable broth and plant-based milk.

Alternatively, mushroom and leek pies, spinach and "cheese" pies, or curried vegetable pies are excellent savory vegan options. To add a finishing touch to these pies, vegan whipped cream made from coconut milk or the liquid from a can of chickpeas can be used as a delicious topping. Sprinkling nuts, seeds, or coconut flakes on top of fruit pies can also enhance their visual appeal and provide additional texture and flavor. Vegan pies not only offer a compassionate and eco-friendly choice but also highlight the versatility and tastiness of plant-based ingredients.

Whether you're looking for a sweet treat or a savory delight, vegan pies are sure to captivate your palate and leave you wanting more. So, the next time you're in the mood for a delectable and guilt-free pie experience, give a vegan pie a try!

Apple pie is a timeless and beloved dessert that holds a special place in the hearts of many around the world. With its flaky crust, tender spiced apples, and comforting aroma, apple pie is a true classic that has been enjoyed for generations. At the heart of every apple pie is, of course, the apples. The choice of apple variety can greatly influence the final taste and texture of the pie.

Some popular apple varieties used in apple pies include Granny Smith, Honeycrisp, Fuji, and Gala. Each apple brings its unique blend of sweetness and tartness, and the best pies often combine different types of apples for a more complex flavor profile. To create the perfect filling, the apples are typically combined with sugar, cinnamon, and a touch of lemon juice or apple cider vinegar to enhance the fruit's natural flavors. Some bakers may also add a pinch of nutmeg or cloves to add extra warmth and depth to the filling. The mixture is then piled into the pie crust, ready to be covered and baked. Speaking of crust, a well-made pie crust is essential to the success of an apple pie.

A classic double-crust is often used, where a bottom crust lines the pie dish, and a top crust covers the apple filling. The crust is typically made from a blend of flour, fat (such as butter or shortening), a little sugar, and ice water to bring it together. The key to a flaky crust is to keep the fat cold and to avoid overworking the dough. Once the pie is assembled, it goes into the oven to bake until the crust is golden brown, and the apples are tender. As it bakes, the tantalizing aroma of cinnamon and baked apples fills the kitchen, creating an irresistible allure.

Apple pie can be served warm or at room temperature, often accompanied by a scoop of vanilla ice cream or a dollop of whipped cream. The contrast of the creamy, cool topping with the warm, fragrant pie is a delightful experience for the senses. In addition to its delicious taste, apple pie also holds a place in cultural and historical significance. It's a symbol of comfort, family gatherings, and celebrations, particularly in American culture where it is often associated with holidays like Thanksgiving. Whether enjoyed on a special occasion or as a simple treat on a cozy evening, apple pie remains a cherished dessert that brings people together and evokes feelings of nostalgia and joy. Its time-honored recipe and heartwarming flavors ensure that apple pie will continue to be a cherished dessert for generations to come.

2.2

The natural sweetness and juiciness of ripe peaches are celebrated in the delicious and unmistakably summertime delicacy known as peach pie. Just like apple pie, it holds a special place in the hearts of dessert lovers around the world, offering a natural sweetness and juiciness of ripe peaches are celebrated in the delicious and unmistakably summertime delicacy known as peach pie. burst of vibrant flavor and a taste of the season's bounty. The star of any peach pie is, of course, the peaches themselves. The ideal peaches for pie-making are those that are ripe yet firm, as they hold their shape well during baking. Varieties like Freestone or Clingstone peaches are commonly used, with their juicy flesh and rich flavor. To prepare the filling, the peaches are peeled, pitted, and sliced. They are then gently tossed with sugar, a splash of lemon juice, and perhaps a pinch of cinnamon or nutmeg to enhance the natural sweetness and add a hint of warmth.

Some bakers may also incorporate cornstarch or tapioca flour to thicken the juices released by the peaches during baking, ensuring a luscious and cohesive filling. The pie crust for a peach pie is usually made using the same principles as for other fruit pies. A buttery and flaky crust provides the perfect canvas for the succulent peach filling. Some bakers might opt for a lattice top crust, allowing the peachy goodness to peek through in a beautiful woven pattern.

Once the pie is assembled, it is baked until the crust turns a golden brown, and the peach filling bubbles with irresistible sweetness. The aroma of the peaches and spices fills the kitchen, beckoning everyone to gather around in eager anticipation. Peach pie can be enjoyed on its own, but it pairs exceptionally well with a scoop of vanilla ice cream or a dollop of whipped cream. The contrast between the warm pie and the cool, creamy topping creates a delightful and satisfying dessert experience. Like many fruit pies, peach pie has cultural significance in various regions. In the southern United States, for example, peach pie is a beloved dessert during the summer months when peaches are in season. It has become a symbol of hospitality and southern charm, often served at gatherings and family gatherings.

Whether you're celebrating a special occasion, hosting a summer barbecue, or simply craving the taste of juicy peaches, peach pie is a wonderful way to indulge in the flavors of the season. It's refreshing taste, heartwarming aroma, and versatility make it a dessert that is sure to bring smiles and joy to those who have the pleasure of savoring it.

2.3

Coconut cream pie is a luscious and decadent dessert that combines the tropical flavors of coconut with a rich and creamy custard filling. This delightful pie is a true indulgence, loved by coconut enthusiasts and dessert connoisseurs alike. At the heart of a coconut cream pie is the velvety custard filling. It is made by gently cooking a mixture of coconut milk, coconut cream, sugar, and egg yolks until it thickens to a smooth and creamy consistency. The coconut milk and cream infuse the custard with a delightful coconut essence, while the egg yolks contribute to its luxurious texture and flavor.

To enhance the tropical coconut experience, some bakers might also add shredded coconut or coconut flakes to the filling. This not only adds a subtle crunch but also intensifies the coconut flavor, creating a true coconut lover's dream. The filling is poured into a pre-baked pie crust, which can be either a traditional buttery pastry crust or a graham cracker crust for a nutty and slightly sweet base. Once assembled, the pie is chilled until the custard sets, allowing the flavors to meld together. Just before serving, the pie is usually topped with a generous layer of whipped cream, which adds a light and airy contrast to the rich coconut custard. The whipped cream can be further garnished with toasted coconut flakes, creating a visually stunning dessert that is as delightful to look at as it is to eat.

Coconut cream pie is perfect for warm weather or any occasion where a tropical flair is desired. Its creamy, coconut-infused filling and sweet, flaky crust make it an irresistible treat that can transport you to a sunny island paradise with each bite.

The dessert's popularity can be attributed to its delightful combination of flavors and textures, making it a beloved choice for potlucks, family gatherings, and special celebrations. Whether enjoyed at home, in a restaurant, or at a holiday feast, coconut cream pie never fails to evoke feelings of indulgence and satisfaction.

For those who appreciate the taste of coconut and crave a dessert that's a little exotic, coconut cream pie is a must-try. Its harmonious blend of coconut, creaminess, and sweetness ensures that it remains a classic favorite among dessert enthusiasts of all ages. So, if you haven't already experienced the joy of coconut cream pie, treat yourself to this tropical delight and savor the taste of paradise.

Chapter 3

Vegan Cakes

Vegan cakes are delicious and compassionate desserts that cater to individuals following a plant-based lifestyle. Since they don't include any components originating from animals, such as eggs, cheese, and honey, they offer a guilty-free treat. Despite the absence of traditional animal-based components, vegan cakes are just as flavorful, moist, and delightful as their non-vegan counterparts.

The foundation of a vegan cake lies in replacing the traditional eggs and dairy with clever plant-based substitutes. For example, ripe mashed bananas, applesauce, silken tofu, or flaxseed mixed with water can act as excellent egg replacements, providing moisture and binding properties. Non-dairy milk, such as almond milk, soy milk, or coconut milk, replaces cow's milk, adding creaminess and enhancing the overall taste. A variety of flours can be used in vegan cakes, including all-purpose flour, whole wheat flour, spelt flour, almond flour, or gluten-free flours for those with dietary restrictions. Combining different types of flour can result in unique textures and flavors.

Vegan cakes come in a wide range of flavors, just like traditional cakes. Classic flavors like vanilla, chocolate, and lemon are popular choices, while more adventurous options like carrot cake, red velvet, or matcha green tea cakes are also gaining popularity.

For the frosting, traditional buttercream is substituted with vegan butter or plant-based spreads. Alternatively, a frosting can be made using coconut cream, avocado, or nut butters for a more wholesome approach. The result is a smooth and delectable frosting that complements the cake perfectly. Vegan cakes are not only compassionate and sustainable choices, but they can also accommodate various dietary restrictions, making them a great option for gatherings where dietary preferences vary. The popularity of vegan cakes has been growing steadily, driven by the increasing interest in plant-based diets and the desire for more ethical and environmentally-friendly food choices. Many bakeries and restaurants now offer a variety of vegan cake options to cater to this growing demand.

Whether you're a vegan or just someone looking to explore new and delicious desserts, vegan cakes are a wonderful choice. With their delectable flavors and moist textures, these plant-based treats are sure to win over the hearts (and taste buds) of anyone who tries them. So, don't hesitate to treat yourself to a slice of vegan cake and discover the delightful world of cruelty-free baking.

3.1

Vanilla cake is a timeless and beloved dessert that captures the delicate essence of pure vanilla. It is a classic choice for many occasions, from birthday celebrations to weddings, and its light, tender crumb and sweet, fragrant flavor make it a universally adored treat. At the heart of a vanilla cake is the star ingredient: vanilla extract. This natural essence is obtained from the beans of the vanilla orchid, imparting a distinct and comforting aroma to the cake. The use of high-quality vanilla extract is essential in creating a cake that truly highlights the unique essence of this cherished spice.

To prepare the batter, a blend of flour, sugar, baking powder, and a pinch of salt is mixed together. Vegan vanilla cake recipes will often call for plant-based milk, such as almond milk or soy milk, and vegetable oil as substitutes for dairy milk and butter, making it suitable for those following a plant-based lifestyle. Traditional recipes may call for milk and butter, which also create a tender and moist texture. Eggs are a common ingredient in traditional vanilla cake recipes, but they can be substituted with vegan alternatives like applesauce, mashed bananas, or commercial egg replacers. These substitutes help bind the ingredients and provide structure to the cake, resulting in a soft and light crumb.

Once the batter is mixed, the fragrant vanilla extract is added, infusing the cake with its warm and comforting aroma. The batter is then poured into cake pans and baked until it turns a golden brown, filling the kitchen with the sweet scent of vanilla.

Vanilla cake can be enjoyed as a simple single-layer cake or a more elaborate layer cake. It is often paired with a velvety vanilla buttercream frosting, which further accentuates the cake's vanilla flavor. Some bakers may add a touch of vanilla bean seeds to the frosting for a visually striking and intensely aromatic effect.

While vanilla cake is delicious on its own, it serves as a versatile canvas for other flavor combinations. It can be complemented with fresh berries, chocolate ganache, or citrus glazes to add extra layers of taste and texture. The simplicity and elegance of vanilla cake have made it a staple in the world of baking. Its universal appeal and ability to accommodate various dietary preferences, including vegan options, have made it a go-to dessert for a wide range of celebrations and gatherings.

Whether it's a special occasion or an ordinary day, a slice of vanilla cake never fails to bring joy and comfort. Its subtle sweetness and comforting aroma create a nostalgic experience that resonates with dessert enthusiasts of all ages, making it a timeless classic that continues to delight and impress.

Chocolate cake is a beloved and indulgent dessert that has been captivating taste buds for generations. Its rich, moist, and chocolatey goodness makes it a perennial favorite at celebrations, gatherings, and as a special treat for any occasion. At the heart of a chocolate cake is, of course, chocolate! Cocoa powder or melted chocolate is incorporated into the batter, giving the cake its deep, decadent flavor. The type and quality of chocolate used can greatly influence the final taste, with options ranging from sweet milk chocolate to intense dark chocolate.

To create the perfect chocolate cake, bakers combine the chocolate with other essential ingredients, such as flour, sugar, eggs, butter (or plant-based alternatives for vegan versions), and buttermilk or sour cream for added moisture and richness. Baking soda or baking powder is used as a leavening agent to ensure a light and airy crumb.

Once the batter is prepared, it is poured into cake pans and baked to perfection. As the cake bakes, the irresistible aroma of chocolate fills the kitchen, making it hard to resist anticipation for the finished creation. Chocolate cake offers endless possibilities for variations and customizations. While a classic chocolate cake is delicious on its own, it can be transformed into a variety of mouthwatering delights.

For example:

Chocolate Layer Cake: Bakers often divide the batter between multiple cake pans to create layers that are sandwiched together with frosting, making for an impressive and indulgent treat.

Chocolate Cupcakes: Portioning the batter into cupcake molds creates adorable and convenient individual servings.

Chocolate Sheet Cake: Baking the batter in a rectangular pan result in a more casual, yet equally delicious, cake that is easy to serve at gatherings.

Flourless Chocolate Cake: For those seeking a gluten-free option, flour can be omitted from the recipe, resulting in a dense and fudgy cake with an intense chocolate flavor.

Chocolate cake can be adorned with a variety of frostings and fillings, such as classic buttercream, cream cheese frosting, ganache, or even chocolate mousse, which adds an extra layer of decadence.

The universal appeal of chocolate cake lies in its ability to evoke feelings of comfort and delight. Whether enjoyed with a glass of cold milk, a hot cup of coffee, or as a dessert after a special meal, chocolate cake never fails to satisfy sweet cravings and put a smile on people of all ages' faces.

From simple family gatherings to elaborate celebrations, chocolate cake remains a timeless and cherished dessert that is sure to please chocolate enthusiasts and dessert lovers alike. So, the next time you're looking to indulge in something sweet and delightful, treat yourself to a slice of heavenly chocolate cake and savor its irresistible allure.

3.3

Carrot cake is a delightful and unique dessert that has gained popularity around the world for its moist, flavorful, and wholesome qualities. Combining the natural sweetness of carrots with warm spices and a luscious cream cheese frosting, carrot cake is a true crowd-pleaser loved by many.

At the core of a carrot cake are grated carrots, which not only provide natural sweetness but also add moisture and texture to the cake. The carrots are combined with a blend of basic ingredients such as flour, sugar, eggs, and oil (or butter for a richer version), along with a medley of warm spices like cinnamon, nutmeg, and cloves. The result is a cake with a tender crumb and a well-balanced taste that tantalizes the taste buds. One of the charms of carrot cake lies in its adaptability. Nuts like chopped walnuts or pecans are often folded into the batter, adding a delightful crunch and nutty flavor. Some bakers may even add shredded coconut or raisins for extra texture and complexity.

Once the batter is prepared, it's poured into cake pans and baked to perfection. As it bakes, the kitchen is filled with the inviting aroma of cinnamon and spices, building anticipation for the scrumptious treat to come. A defining feature of carrot cake is its cream cheese frosting, which complements the earthy flavors of the cake with a creamy and tangy sweetness. The frosting is made by combining cream cheese, butter, powdered sugar, and vanilla extract. The smooth and velvety texture of the cream cheese frosting adds a luxurious touch, making carrot cake all the more delectable.

Carrot cake can be enjoyed in various forms, such as a classic layer cake, cupcakes, or even a sheet cake. Its versatility extends to its presentation, with some cakes adorned with delicate carrot decorations or chopped nuts on top, adding a visual appeal that matches its enticing taste. Beyond its delectable flavor, carrot cake has some healthful attributes. The addition of carrots provides essential nutrients and fiber, making it a dessert that's slightly more guilt-free than some other indulgences.

Carrot cake's popularity continues to grow as more people appreciate its unique blend of flavors and textures. Whether served at family gatherings, celebrations, or simply as a treat for yourself, carrot cake remains a beloved and cherished dessert that never fails to bring smiles to faces and warmth to hearts. So, the next time you're seeking a sweet and satisfying treat, give in to the allure of carrot cake and enjoy its delightful fusion of sweet and spiced goodness.

Chapter 4

Vegan Cheesecake

Vegan cheesecake is a delightful and creamy dessert that captures the essence of traditional cheesecake while adhering to a plant-based lifestyle. Made without any animal-derived ingredients like cream cheese and eggs, this dairy-free version is perfect for vegans and those looking for a lighter and more ethical dessert option. The key to creating a luscious vegan cheesecake lies in finding suitable substitutes for the classic ingredients. Instead of dairy cream cheese, vegan bakers often use cashews as the base for the filling. Soaked and blended cashews create a wonderfully smooth and creamy texture that mimics the richness of traditional cheesecake. To enhance the flavor and tanginess that cream cheese provides, lemon juice or apple cider vinegar is added to the cashew mixture. This addition not only adds a pleasant zing but also replicates the characteristic tang of cheesecake. To sweeten the filling, bakers typically use a combination of natural sweeteners like maple syrup, agave nectar, or coconut sugar. These alternatives provide the right amount of sweetness without relying on refined sugars or honey.

The crust for vegan cheesecake can be made in various ways. A classic graham cracker crust can be easily used as vegan graham crackers and dairy-free butter. Alternatively, crushed nuts, coconut flakes, or dates can be used to create a crust that complements the flavors of the creamy filling. Once the filling is blended to perfection, it is poured into the prepared crust and refrigerated to set. The chilling process allows the flavors to meld together and the texture to become firmer, creating a cheesecake-like consistency. Vegan cheesecake offers a canvas for a wide range of flavors and variations. You can infuse the filling with additional ingredients like cocoa powder for a chocolate twist or fresh fruit puree for a fruity burst. Toppings like berry compote, chocolate ganache, or crushed nuts can further enhance the cheesecake's visual appeal and taste.

The versatility and delectable taste of vegan cheesecake have made it a beloved dessert among vegans and non-vegans alike. It offers a guilt-free and compassionate indulgence that aligns with ethical and environmental principles.

Whether you're a vegan seeking a decadent treat or someone simply looking to explore new dessert options, vegan cheesecake is a delightful and satisfying choice. So, next time you're craving a creamy and dreamy dessert, try a slice of vegan cheesecake and savor the creamy goodness without any animal products.

New York-style cheesecake is a legendary and iconic dessert that has become synonymous with rich, velvety texture and a classic taste. Originating from the Big Apple, this cheesecake has garnered a massive fan following worldwide for its indulgent and decadent qualities.

The hallmark of New York-style cheesecake is its dense and creamy filling, which sets it apart from other cheesecake variations. The base ingredients usually include cream cheese, eggs, sugar, and heavy cream. The cream cheese is the star of the show, providing the cake with its unmistakable smoothness and tanginess. To prepare the filling, bakers start by beating the cream cheese until it's light and fluffy. Then, they incorporate the sugar, eggs, and heavy cream, ensuring a perfectly smooth and cohesive mixture. The use of heavy cream adds an extra level of richness, making this cheesecake the epitome of luxurious indulgence.

Another critical aspect of a New York-style cheesecake is the crust. A classic graham cracker crust is often used, made from a combination of crushed graham crackers, sugar, and melted butter. This crust provides a delightful contrast to the creamy filling, adding a crisp and slightly sweet base to the cake. Once the crust and filling are combined, the cheesecake is baked at a low temperature until it's set but still has a slight jiggle in the center. The slow baking process helps prevent cracks and ensures the cheesecake retains its signature velvety texture.

New York-style cheesecake is often served plain, allowing the simple yet luxurious flavors of the cream cheese to shine through. However, it's also a versatile canvas for a variety of toppings and variations. Some popular options include fresh fruit compote, chocolate ganache, caramel sauce, or a dusting of powdered sugar. When enjoying a slice of New York-style cheesecake, you'll experience the decadence of each mouthful. The velvety, creamy texture combined with the slight tang of cream cheese creates an unforgettable and truly indulgent dessert experience.

New York-style cheesecake has become a fixture in bakeries and dessert menus worldwide, and its reputation continues to grow. Whether you're in the heart of New York City or on the other side of the globe, this classic dessert is sure to captivate your taste buds and leave you longing for just one more heavenly bite.

Strawberry cheesecake is a delightful and luscious dessert that combines the rich creaminess of cheesecake with the sweet and tangy flavors of fresh strawberries. This delectable treat is a favorite among dessert enthusiasts, offering a delightful taste of summer in every bite. At the heart of strawberry cheesecake is the creamy and velvety cheesecake filling. Cream cheese is combined with eggs, sugar, and vanilla extract to create the base. The cream cheese provides the cake with its iconic smooth and rich texture, while the eggs help bind the ingredients together and create a stable structure.

To incorporate the strawberries, a fresh strawberry puree or chopped strawberries are folded into the cheesecake filling. The natural sweetness and tartness of the strawberries complement the creamy base, creating a harmonious balance of flavors. The crust for strawberry cheesecake is usually a classic graham cracker crust, made from crushed graham crackers, sugar, and melted butter. The crisp and slightly sweet crust offers a delightful contrast to the creamy filling and juicy strawberries. Once the filling is combined with the crust, the cheesecake is baked until it's set and has a slight jiggle in the center. After baking, it's important to let the cheesecake cool and then refrigerate it for several hours or overnight to allow the flavors to meld together and for the cheesecake to become firm.

When serving strawberry cheesecake, it's customary to add a topping of fresh strawberries. The bright red strawberries add a burst of color and freshness to the dessert, enhancing its visual appeal and taste. Strawberry cheesecake is perfect for warm weather or any occasion where a burst of fruity goodness is desired. It's a wonderful addition to summer parties, picnics, and celebrations, bringing a taste of the season's bounty to the table. This dessert has a universal appeal, loved by both kids and adults alike. Its creamy, tangy, and fruity flavors make it an all-time favorite that never fails to impress.

Whether you're a cheesecake lover or a strawberry enthusiast, strawberry cheesecake is sure to captivate your taste buds with its irresistible combination of textures and flavors. So, the next time you're craving a delightful and refreshing dessert, treat yourself to a slice of strawberry cheesecake and savor the joy of each delightful bite.

Key Lime cheesecake is a delectable and zesty dessert that marries the lusciousness of cheesecake with the refreshing tang of Key lime flavor. This delightful treat is a perfect fusion of tropical and creamy goodness, bringing a taste of the Florida Keys to dessert tables around the world. At the heart of Key Lime cheesecake is the rich and creamy cheesecake filling, typically made with cream cheese, eggs, sugar, and a hint of vanilla extract. The cream cheese provides the cake with its velvety texture, while the eggs help bind the ingredients together and create a stable structure. To infuse the cheesecake with the iconic Key lime flavor, freshly squeezed Key lime juice and grated zest are added to the filling. Key limes are smaller and more tart than regular limes, which gives the cheesecake a uniquely tangy and vibrant taste. The crust for Key Lime cheesecake is usually a classic graham cracker crust, made from crushed graham crackers, sugar, and melted butter. The sweet and slightly crunchy crust perfectly complements the creamy filling and zesty lime flavors.

Once the filling is combined with the crust, the cheesecake is baked until it's set and has a slight jiggle in the center. After baking, it's important to let the cheesecake cool and then refrigerate it for several hours or overnight to allow the flavors to meld together and for the cheesecake to become firm. When serving Key Lime cheesecake, it's customary to add a topping of whipped cream or a dollop of lime curd. The light and airy whipped cream or the sweet-tart lime curd add an extra layer of flavor and texture to the dessert, elevating it to a whole new level of indulgence.

Key Lime cheesecake is perfect for warm weather or any occasion where a refreshing and tropical dessert is desired. Its bright and zesty flavors make it a wonderful addition to summer gatherings, beach parties, and celebrations.

This dessert has a unique and invigorating appeal, loved by those who appreciate the bold and refreshing taste of Key lime. Whether you're a fan of traditional cheesecake or a lover of all things citrusy, Key Lime cheesecake is sure to captivate your taste buds and transport you to a sunny and tropical paradise with each delightful bite. So, the next time you're looking for a delightful and zesty dessert that's full of tropical flair, treat yourself to a slice of Key Lime cheesecake and savor the blissful combination of creamy and tangy goodness.

CONCLUSION

In conclusion, a vegan dessert cookbook is not just a collection of recipes; it is a celebration of the extraordinary possibilities that lie within the realm of vegan desserts. Throughout these pages, we have embarked on a delightful culinary journey, exploring the rich tapestry of flavors, textures, and ingredients that plant-based baking has to offer. In creating this cookbook, our primary goal was to show that vegan desserts are far from limiting or bland; rather, they open up a world of creativity and innovation. From the simplicity of vegan classics revamped to the decadence of chocolate delights, the tropical inspirations that transport us to sun-kissed shores, and the nutty indulgences that awaken our taste buds, we have curated a diverse and exciting range of desserts to cater to every palate and occasion.

One of the most remarkable aspects of vegan desserts is their ability to accommodate various dietary preferences and restrictions. With recipes that are free from dairy, eggs, and animal-derived ingredients, these treats can be enjoyed by vegans and those with dairy allergies, lactose intolerance, or ethical considerations. Moreover, they offer a healthier alternative for those looking to reduce their intake of refined sugars and unhealthy fats, without sacrificing on taste or satisfaction.

Throughout the creation of this cookbook, we have sought to showcase the immense potential of plant-based ingredients and their ability to elevate desserts to new heights. The delicate confections demonstrate the elegance and artistry that can be achieved through vegan baking, proving that dessert-making can be an expression of both culinary skill and love for the environment and animals. Additionally, the chapter on healthier bites showcases that desserts need not always be indulgent in a traditional sense, but can still offer moments of comfort and joy through nourishing and wholesome ingredients. These treats are a reminder that self-care can manifest through the act of creating and savoring foods that nurture the body and soul.

At the core of this cookbook is a commitment to sustainability, compassion, and a better future for our planet. By choosing to explore the world of vegan desserts, we actively contribute to reducing our carbon footprint, conserving natural resources, and fostering a kinder and more ethical relationship with the world around us. As we come to the end of this culinary voyage, we hope you have found inspiration, joy, and a deeper appreciation for the beauty of vegan desserts. We encourage you to take these recipes and make them your own, adapting and experimenting to suit your tastes and preferences. Whether you're a seasoned vegan or a curious food enthusiast, may these recipes serve as a stepping stone into a world of compassionate and mouthwatering dessert creations.

Thank you for joining us on this delightful journey of discovery. May you continue to embrace the incredible potential of plant-based baking and find joy in the process of creating and sharing these Plant-Based Delights with your loved ones. Here's to a sweeter, more compassionate world, one delicious bite at a time.

Happy baking!